Demystifying Cancer

Other titles in Sede Series

PEDRO-SALVADOR Abdulateef: Demystifying Cancer (The Predisposing Factors)
PEDRO-SALVADOR Abdulateef: Educine: Educal Studies For Teaching
PEDRO-SALVADOR Abdulateef: Tabularasa: The Repository of Learning
PEDRO-SALVADOR Abdulateef: Modern Genetic Inheritance (Mendelian) Vol. 1
PEDRO-SALVADOR Abdulateef: Modern Genetic Inheritance (Mathematical Version) Vol. 2
PEDRO-SALVADOR Abdulateef: Modern Genetic Inheritance (Compendium of Discovery, Invention, Hypotheses, Innovations and Rules)
PEDRO-SALVADOR Abdulateef: Introduction to Genetic Inheritance

Demystifying Cancer

The Predisposing Factors

Pedro-Salvador Abdulateef *(Certified Teacher)*

BSc (Education) Physics (Uinlag), NCE Chemistry/Physics(Unilag), OND Elect. &
Elect. Eng; (YCT)

Sede School of Educine, Lagos, Nigeria.
Educal Studies

Publisher: Muhammad Pedro
Copy Editor: Muhammad Olayiwola Pedro
Photo Researcher: Pedro Media
Images: Pixabay.com, Pedro Media
Page layout: Pedro Media

First Published 2018

ISBN: 9781717792723

Preface

The purpose of this book is to:

I. Create awareness about the origin, root, causes and precursor of CANCER
II. Educate the populace about the factors, habits and lifestyles that predispose one of the risks of cancer.
III. Enlighten individuals on the meaning of (I) Mutation (II) Metastasis (III) Tumor and (IV) Cancer.
IV. Attempt to present to the masses irrespective of the level of education sensitization tactics in form of three series of writing: SERIES ONE, SERIES TWO AND SERIES THREE.

SERIES ONE: for the use of layman and primary learners.

SERIES TWO: for the scholars and secondary learners.

SERIES THREE: for the intellectuals and stakeholders.

Table of Contents

Programme 1

Cancer is a consequence of a faulty gene. Genes are located in human (system) body. Touch your skin, prick it and pull it up. That part of your body is an example of an organ. There are several organs in human body: Breast, Cervix, Eye, Ailment, Kidney, Liver, Lungs, Blood and so on.

An organ is made of two or more types of *tissue* of different kinds. A tissue is composed of cells of the same kind. A cell contains Protoplasm and *nucleus*. In the nucleus are chromosomes. On each chromosome are located genes. *so genes*

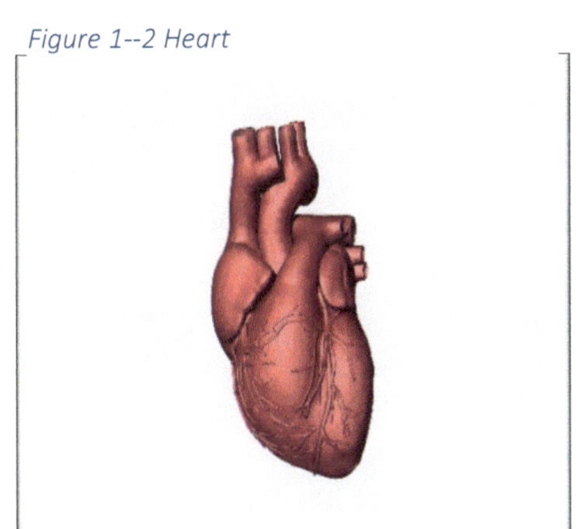

Figure 1--2 Heart

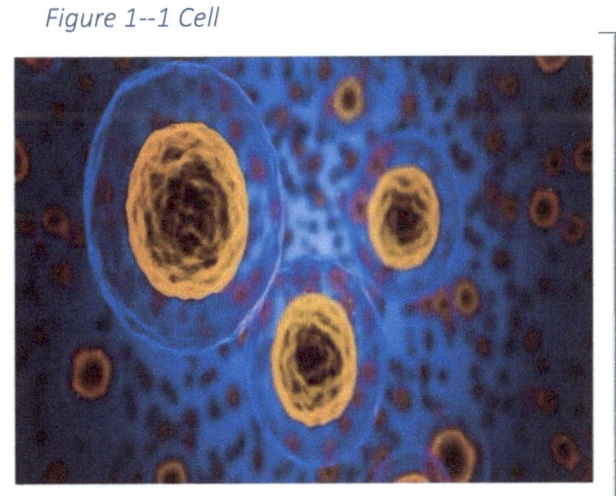

Figure 1--1 Cell

are inside our body, genes are everywhere, all over our body

The diagrams above are examples of organs and Cell. Cells are extremely tiny and may not be seen ordinarily. However, *a hen's egg* is an example of a sex-cell. The yoke of an egg is the *nucleus*. The albumen is the cytoplasm, so to say. In the yoke are *chromosomes*. On the *chromosomes* are the *genes* located so every cell in our body like an *egg* is, an *egg* is a sex cell but body cell is called the Somatic cell.

Sex cell reproduces by copulation, meiosis fertilization and Divisions. *somatic* cell reproduces by *replication* and Divisions. What causes or prompt Division of cell? It is the *gene, gene gives instructions,* before you go further on this programme read this passage two or more times again, for better understanding. Note the keywords, and new terms. Write them down.

Practice Question 1.

1) Explain the following in your own words: (i) SYSTEM (ii) BODY (iii) ORGAN (iv) CELL.
2) What is the difference between (a) a sex cell and (b) somatic cell?
3) Which type of cell is readily available in the market?

Practice Question 2.

Fill in the gaps.

In the human body, --A-- are located to control biological process. —B-- consists of cell wall, protoplasm, nucleus, among others. —C—is a part of human body that is made up of a number of different TISSUES specialized to carry out a particular function. Fowl's egg is an example of a ----D-----

----

Answer.

A. *(GENES)* B. *(CELL)*   C. *(ORGAN)*   D. *(CELL)*

How many of these questions did you get right? If your total score is below 50%. Repeat programme 1 again, otherwise move to programme 2.

Worksheet 1

Programme 2

A gene is a biological logic device; a logic device is one that has its specific form of language. A language is a special means of communication. Communication is a means of transmitting information or message from one point to another point.

Logic is a sort of operation, just as mathematics is a form of another operation. Alphanumeric is another form of operation that combines two forms of operation.

Alphabetic operation and numeric operation. Logic also has some forms of operation. (a) Binary (b) Ternary (c) Quaternary among other operations

Practice Question 3.

Fill in the gaps.

Language is a form of operation just like mathematics is a form of —E—English is a form of operation just like Chinese is another form of —F—Arabic is a peculiar form of operation just like Greek has its own peculiar form of —G—Chinese, Greek, Arabic, Mathematics and logic are all forms of —H—Therefore a language is an —I—having its characteristics.

Answer.

E. (OPERATION)   F. (OPERATION) G. (OPERATION)
H. (OPERATION)   I. (OPERATION)

Operation means a function, working activity or manner in which something functions. Language means a form of code. A form of code in Greek is different for that of Chinese, Arabic or Latin. Since the *coding* systems in these four languages are different from one another, they are called classical language. Code is a specialized or private *language* of communication. Logic is the process of operating a code system.

In electronics, transistors and diodes are the logic devices, in biology Nucleic acids are the logic devices, electronic logic devices have logic functions and operations. Biological logic devices have their logic functions and operations different that of electronic system.

Logic devices code a message and communicate from one point to the other. Interestingly all living creatures are in groups and members of each group communicate with one another in their *(code)* language.

Birds have their own *(code)* language fishes have their code or language different from that of frogs or lions or ants or spider. Bees have interesting code system. Even the deaf and dumb communicate in code.

So animal's biology (especially human) has a code (language) system whose means of operation is *logic*. So *logic* is a process of operating a code, so GENE is human logic device system that operates biology logic code for communication.

Physiological processes in biology are carried out by means of logic operations. Digestion, Metabolism, Fertilization, Meiosis, Breathing Respiration, Dialysis and several other are all logic operations consequence.

Growth, Excretion, Healing, Repair, and other are all consequences of logic operation communicated by the *genes*, so genes are the logic Devices and are composed of *nucleic acids*.

Practice Question 4.

Fill in the gaps.
Code system is a form of language system, and language is a form of -----J---. Greek is a form of ----K----- or -----------L----------- designed by the Greek. ----M---- is a form of ------N------ designed by the Chinese, Ancient ARABS designed ------O---- In ARABIC to help in ----P--- with the world. Genetic code is a form of ---------Q-------- that is used in biological processes

---

Answer.

J. *(CODE)*   K. *(LANGUAGE)*   L. *(CODE)*   M. *(CHINESE)*   N. *(CODE)*
O. *(CODE SYSTEM)*   P. *(COMMUNICATION)*   Q. *(LANGUAGE)*
R. *(GENE)*   S. *(GENES)*

Practice Question 5.

Digestion is a form of logic function instructed by the ----**R**----. Fertilization or growth is a logical operation communicated through ---**S**--- to other organs.

Practice Question 6.

1. What is logic?
2. What is mathematic?
3. Name two forms of universal operation.
4. What is logic element in electronics?
5. What is logic element in biology?
6. What is logic device in electronics?
7. What is logic device in biology?

Answer.

7.*(GENE)*   6. *(INTEGRATED CIRCUIT)*   5. *(NUCLEIC ACID)*   4. *(DIODE AND TRANSISTOR, RESISTOR)*   3. *(MATHEMATICS AND LOGICS)*
2.*(AN OPERATION)*   1. *(AN OPERATION)*

Practice Question 7.

Answer questions (8), (9) and (10) with a diagram.
8. What is cell in biology?

9.   What is protoplasm?
10. What is nucleus?
11. Where are chromosomes located?
12. Where are genes located?
13.   What are the net constituents of a gene?
14.   what are these (i) Acetic acid (II) Nucleic acid
15.   Give one example of an organic acid
16.   What is free Radical?

Answer.
11. (INSIDE THE NUCLEUS) 12. (ON THE CHROMOSOMES) 13. (NUCLEIC ACIDS)
14. (ORGANIC ACIDS) 15. (URIC ACID, FATTY ACID OR AMINO ACID ETCETERA)
16. (IT INITIATES A CHEMICAL REACTION)

Practice Question 8.

Answer the following questions, and score yourself. If you get 75% and above, go to the next programme, otherwise start all over again from programme 1.
1.   What is logic?
2.   What is language?
3.   What is communication?
4.   What is logic element?
5.   What is Electronic logic gate?
6.   What is biological logic gate?
7.   What is Nucleic acid in terms of logic function?
8.   What is semiconductor device in terms of logic function?
9.   What is code?
10. What is gene in terms of language and communication?
11. What is chromosome?
12. What is DNA?
13. What is RNA?
14. What is free Radical?
15. What is a biological logic device?

Practice Question 9.

Complete these statements.
Biology is the science of -----------*A*------------- Human cell consists of --------*B*----
---, protoplasm, ----*C*------ and organelles. The body of human is an assemble of --
------*D*------. Life exists in -------E------- only. Activities of human are due to the
activities its ------*F*------ only Growth of human occurs by cellular growth
or multiplication. There is a relationship between the structure and function
of -----*G*----- is one of the chemical units of hereditary information, found at a
certain location on a ------*H*----, that is responsible for the transmission of
information from one generation to the next Each -----*I*----- contributes to a
particular characteristic of the organism.

Answer.
    I. (GENE)   *H. (CHROMOSOME)*   *G. (GENE)*   *F. (GENE)*
        E. (CELLS)   *D. (CELLS)*   *C. (MEMBRANE)*
        B. (NUCLEUS)   *A. (LIVING THINGS)*

If you score below 75% start from programme 1 again it is important you
understand this section well before you proceed further. Try, don't be
discouraged it is a matter of repetition. You will soon grasp it. It is easy!

Worksheet 2

Worksheet 2

Worksheet 2

Programme 3

Gene is a logic device that uses code for communication to determine hereditary character of organisms including human. Gene is a logic device composed of nucleic acids whose means of transmitting information or messages is in CODE to determine the feature, structure, function and condition of all the tissues and organs of the animals and plant's body. The diagram is an attempt to represent a gene as an illustration. It is a combination of three nucleic acids. It is contained in every cell of the human body. It communicates or determines how the structure of the tissues

Figure 3-1- Illustration of a gene

should be formed, what the feature should look like and how the tissues and the proteins should function. Summarily *gene* determines the *structure, function and condition* of our body.

Gene is composed of Ribose nucleic acids and e oxyribose nucleic acid, RNA and DNA respectively. These two forms of nucleic acids are nothing but giant organic molecules, they are subjected to all chemical rules, laws, and reactions. They can decompose and recompose. Similarly, all material substances

Figure 3-2 De Oxyribose Nucleic Acid

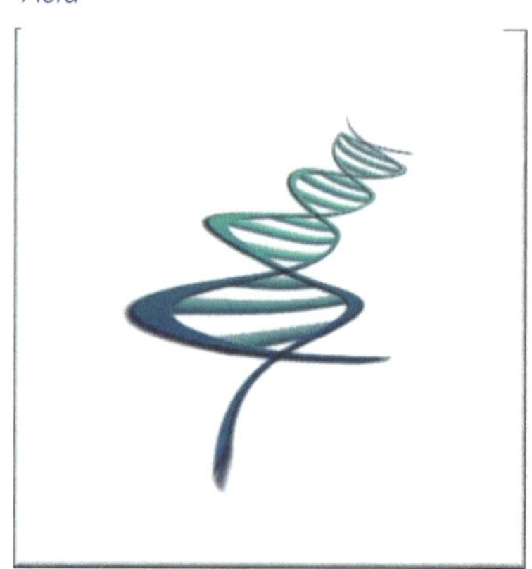

are chemical including water and entire food items, each the following can influence the way the *gene,* a biological logic device work or function. Certain substances including food items and drinks are *inimical* to the gene, the logic device. For example, the *carbon* in smoking is inimical to genes contained in cells or tissue that make up the air passage in human system. Certain condiments or additives contain free radicals that are inimical to the function of Gene, the logic device. There is no end to such a list of extraneous substances

The chemistry of Gene depends on some factors and once the factors are violated, the function of Gene will be disrupted and the genes start to function *wrongly.*

These factors include
1.   Chemical reaction type
2.   Free radical as an initiator of reaction
3.   Destructive Radiation
4.   Habituation or Addiction determining the quantity of reactants in the body.

Mutation Process and Cancer

Naturally or Spontaneously GENE replicates before cell division as shown below.

Figure X-The gene before replication

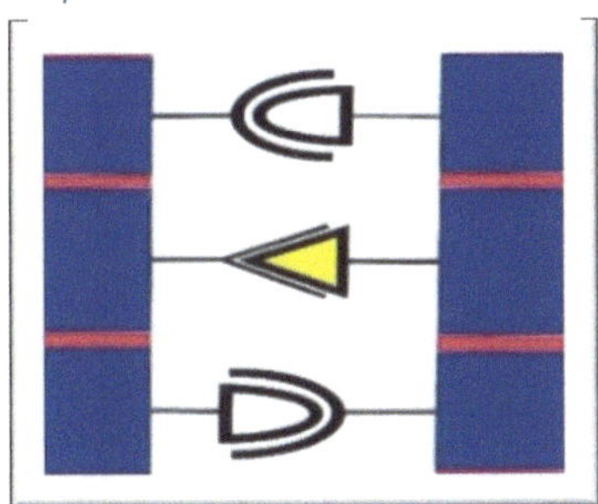

Figure Y-The gene during replication process

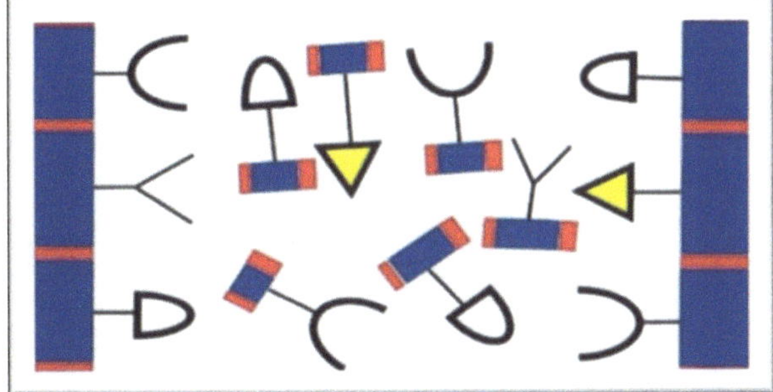

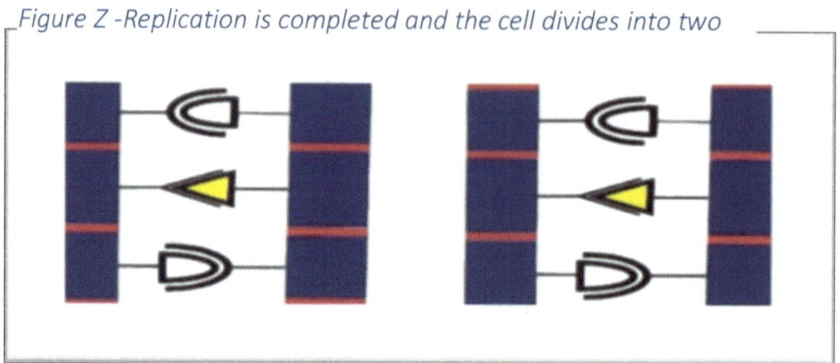

Figure Z -Replication is completed and the cell divides into two

Induced Decomposition and Mutation

Figure P- Normal gene before induced decomposition

Figure Q- Induced decomposition of gene into random nucleotides

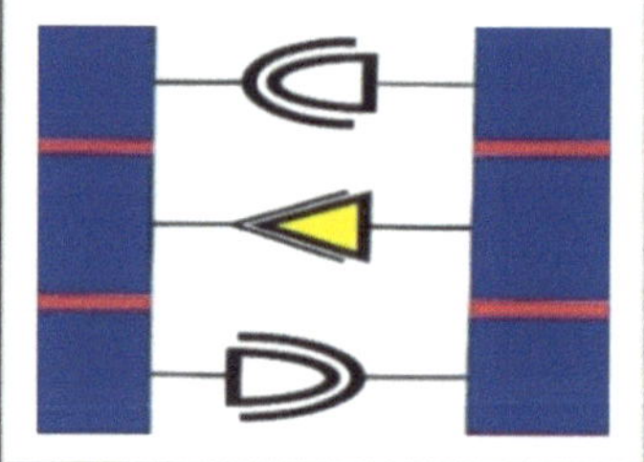

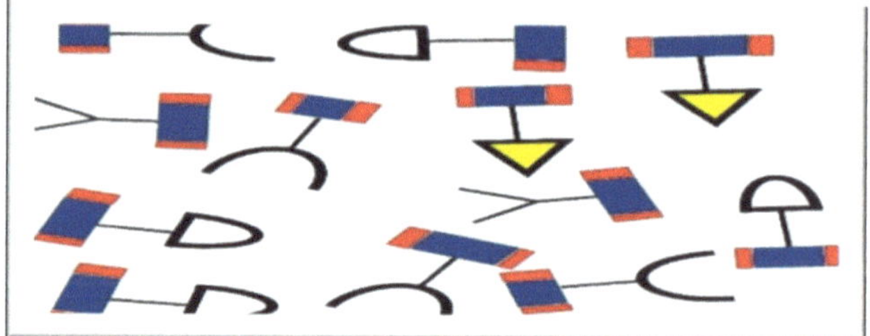

Mutation of Gene

Figure R- Mutation result in formation of two abnormal gene(a) and (b)

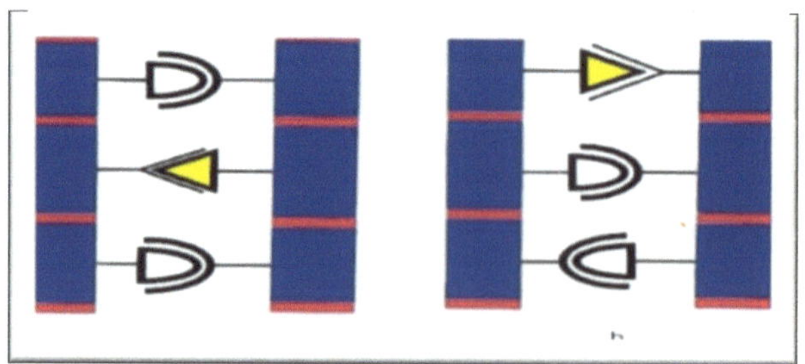

The normal gene (as shown in Fig x) has mutated into two different genes of different sequences of arrangement of the nucleic acids. Fig X. is arbitrarily denoted the normal gene that codes for the normal function of metabolism and other physiological functions. Fig z. is the illustration of replication into two *normal* Genes. This is healthy. Fig r is the illustration of mutation into two *abnormal* Genes. Fig R. (a) and Fig R. (b) This is unhealthy.

Since gene is a logic device, Fig x. codes for normal function, Fig z. also codes for normal function and structure. Fig R (a) and Fig R (b) code for *abnormal function, structure and condition.*

Benign and Malignant Tumor

When abnormal function of genes affects the rate of function of metabolism, the size of the tissues or cells formed is either smaller or bigger than the normal size. This bigger size is often noticed as *tumor*. It may be malignant or benign depending on the organ involved and the impact on the neighboring neutrons.

When the structure or feature only is affected, it may result to other ailments: *Skin cancer, Diabetes, Hypertension, Rheumatism, Arthritis, Cirrhosis, Skin disorder, Dermatitis, Keloid, Moles, Lumps, Vitiligo, Gangrene Xanthelasma, Basal cell Carcinoma and several other non-pathogenic diseases.* It is worth to know that all these ailments mentioned are not *cancer* per se but a sign of approach of permanent *mutation.*

If these signs are noticed in good term and the factor causing them are removed by (A) *Quitting* (B) *Withdrawing* from the *habits* causing them, they will heal and the threat of approaching cancer is nullified.

These factors are
(1) Cosmic Ray Radiation.
(2) Man-made Radiation.
(3) Free Radicals in Sweet Foods and Drinks.
(4) Other Chemical Products.
(5) Quantity (Dosage) of these factors predicated on Habits and Addiction.

The presence of all these at the same time on one particular person predicts the coming of (a) Benign or (b) Malignant *cancer.*

Most of these ailments are signs and symptoms of approaching permanent *mutation*: Prostate enlargement, eczema, high blood pressure, liver diseases, alcoholism all forms of addiction and habituation and several others.

Precaution:

(I) Listen to your body.

(II) Be wary of lifestyle.
(III) Be cautious of your habits: habituation.
(IV) Take only ORGANIC FOODS.

Prevention:

(a) Learn how to withdraw from a suspected habit.
(b) Learn to *quit* a bad habit and addiction.
(c) Minimize your exposure to sun and other forms of ultraviolet, X-ray and Gamma ray, radiations and others.
(d) Do not induce your genetics materials to decomposition.

Metastasis and Habits

When a habit is formed to habituation a human says I cannot do without this or without that. This is a sign of approaching mutation and metastasis. It means extrinsic (new) genes are being formed in some of the cells or tissues all over the body. There are trillions upon trillions of individual cells in human body. It is not all of them that can "share in the impurities or mutagents" simultaneously. Initially very few mutate because the mutagents or impurities cannot go round with time *(habitation or addition)* regular supply is available and more cells or tissues are supplied and eventually the genes there in are mutated. It is this gradual increase in supply of mutagents through habituation and addiction that causes the spread of *mutation* in all the cells and this is known as *metastasis*.

Suggested Solution/Measures

1) Let the victim learn withdrawal method from habituation or addiction.
2) Let the victim learn *quitting* the habit methods.
3) Let the human adopt organic foods habit.
4) And any other specialists' methods.

Worksheet 3